Anticipating The Journey: Insights For Expecting Parents.

Judith R. Price

INTRODUCTION... 3
A: EMBRACING THE WONDERFUL PATH OF
PARENTHOOD... 3
CHAPTER 1.. 10
CHAPTER 2.. 16
CHAPTER 3.. 27
CHAPTER 4.. 36
CHAPTER 5.. 46
CHAPTER 6.. 53
CHAPTER 7.. 62
CHAPTER 8.. 70
CHAPTER 9.. 78
CHAPTER 10.. 87
CONCLUSION..96

INTRODUCTION

A: EMBRACING THE WONDERFUL PATH OF PARENTHOOD

Being a parent is a life-changing and inspiring experience. You are starting a magnificent adventure as expectant parents, one that is accompanied by excitement, joy, and a strong sense of duty. The birth of a child provides unfathomable joy and fulfillment as well as the chance to nurture and direct a priceless existence. It is a journey that offers numerous opportunities for tenderness, development, and learning.

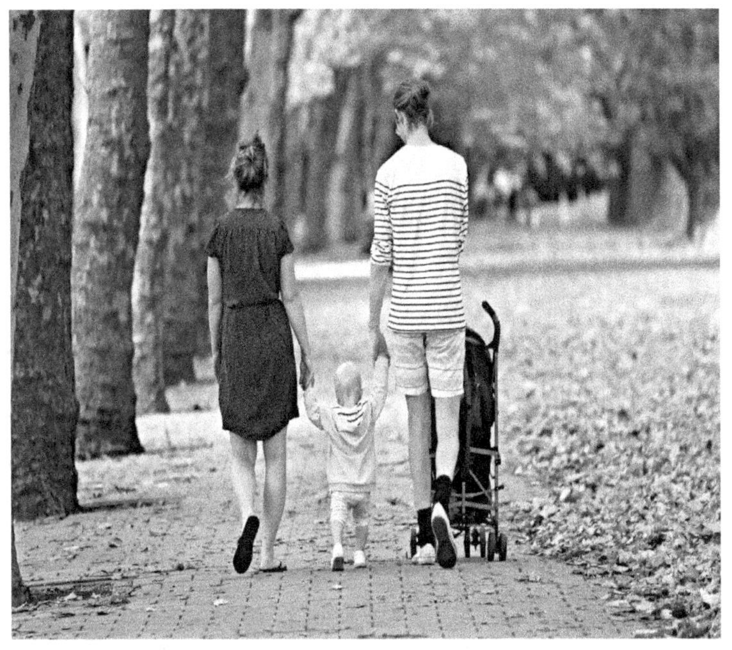

B: The book's goal is to offer advice and thoughts on nurturing

Our goal in "Anticipating the Journey: Nurturing Insights for Expecting Parents" is to walk alongside you on this amazing journey, providing insightful advice and supportive support as you get ready to welcome your child. This book is intended to be your dependable friend, offering comforting assistance during the many phases of pregnancy, childbirth, and early motherhood.

We will go over important subjects in each chapter to give you the tools you need to go on this trip with assurance and delight. We explore the rewards and difficulties of parenting, assisting you in developing a positive outlook and creating a community of like-minded parents. We stress the importance of developing a solid parent-child relationship and offer doable methods for creating love, security, and connection.

We acknowledge the alterations your body experiences during pregnancy, appreciate the wondrous changes, and provide self-care techniques that encourage physical wellness and body acceptance. We also discuss the significance of providing a secure and caring environment for your child and provide helpful advice on arranging a warm and inviting room while putting their safety first.

We talk about budgeting for your expanding family, financial issues, and organizing infant needs, so we do not ignore the practical aspects. Your focus shifts to finding a balance between job and family obligations, enabling you to master the demands of motherhood.

We explore birth options, making a birth plan, and packing necessary items for a pleasant hospital stay as we get ready for the arrival of your little one. We embrace the joy and awe that come with this incredible time as you set off on the adventure of having a baby.

It is important to treasure the first few weeks you have with your baby. To help you through the transition, we give advice on creating routines, fostering moments of bonding, and engaging in self-compassion throughout the postpartum period.

As your child develops, we celebrate their developmental achievements and offer advice on how to comprehend their developmental phases and take part in enriching activities that encourage learning. Taking care of your relationship becomes crucial, and we discuss how to communicate effectively, manage parenting responsibilities, and foster moments of connection and joy.

We highlight the value of self-care for parents during this transforming journey, understanding the relevance of putting your own health first. In addition to offering coping mechanisms for parental stress and weariness, we promote self-compassion and the need for support when necessary.

Take a minute to consider the amazing journey you are about to go on as we draw to a close this book. In closing, we want to encourage you and reassure you that you have love and strength inside of you. Furthermore, we give you access to resources for additional reading and helpful groups, ensuring that you have a wealth of knowledge and networks to support you on your parenting adventure.

With "Anticipating the Journey: Nurturing Insights for Expecting Parents" as your guide, may you discover the motivation, certainty, and resources need to start on this wonderful adventure of parenthood while cherishing each moment and providing your child with unending love and care.

CHAPTER 1

EMBRACING PARENTHOOD

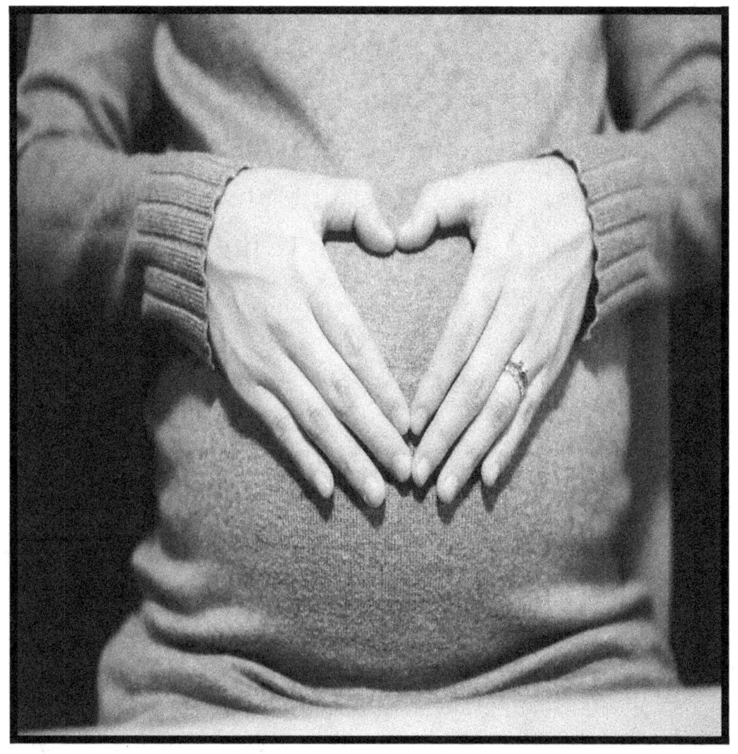

A: Recognizing the Joy and Excitement of Becoming Parents

Being a parent is a very unique and profoundly transformative experience. It's vital to take a minute while you excitedly await the birth of your child to acknowledge the great joy and anticipation that come with this life-changing adventure. Your heart is filled with love, excitement, and amazement as you wait to meet your new baby.

In this chapter, we invite you to cherish the lovely moments of anticipation as you get ready to start this amazing parenting journey. Spend some time appreciating the wonder of life that is developing inside of you and the relationship that has already developed between you and your unborn child. Enjoy the happiness that arises from the idea of holding them in your arms, catching their first grin, and being a guiding force in their lives.

B: Developing a Positive Attitude for the Future

For expectant parents, developing a positive outlook is crucial for overcoming obstacles and appreciating the rewards that lie ahead. A foundation of resilience, hope, and optimism can be built by cultivating a positive mindset while you navigate the ups and downs of parenthood.

Focus on the amazing opportunities for growth and learning that are in store for you as you embrace the positive energy. Develop a mindset that appreciates each accomplishment, treasures each special moment, and finds courage in the face of difficulty. As you begin this new chapter in your life, have faith in your ability to adapt, acquire new skills, and develop alongside your child.

C: Establishing a Community of Like-Minded Parents for Support

Being a parent is not supposed to be an isolated experience. Creating a caring network of other parents can be a priceless source of solace, advice, and fellowship. You can share triumphs, ask for guidance, and take comfort in knowing that you are not alone when you are surrounded by people who are sympathetic to and understand the special experiences of parenthood.

Look for opportunities to interact with other parents in your neighborhood or on websites that encourage expectant parents. Create connections with people who are on this amazing adventure with you by having talks, going to support groups, and taking parenting programs. You may establish a network of support that will be there to encourage, inspire, and provide direction whenever you need it by connecting with people who are familiar with the rewards and difficulties of parenthood.

Keep in mind that every parent's path is different, and there is no one method that works for everyone. Accept the variety of experiences and viewpoints present in your community since it will help you develop a deeper understanding of parenthood. Keep in mind that you have a network of people to lean on and celebrate with as you travel and treasure the times you share laughter, empathy, and encouragement.

Take the time to acknowledge the great delight and anticipation that come with this life-changing experience as you embrace parenting. Develop an optimistic outlook that will enable you to face difficulties with resiliency and hope. Create a welcoming community of other parents, knowing that their compassion and wisdom will be priceless on this wonderful journey of motherhood.

CHAPTER 2

FOSTERING THE PARENT-CHILD BOND

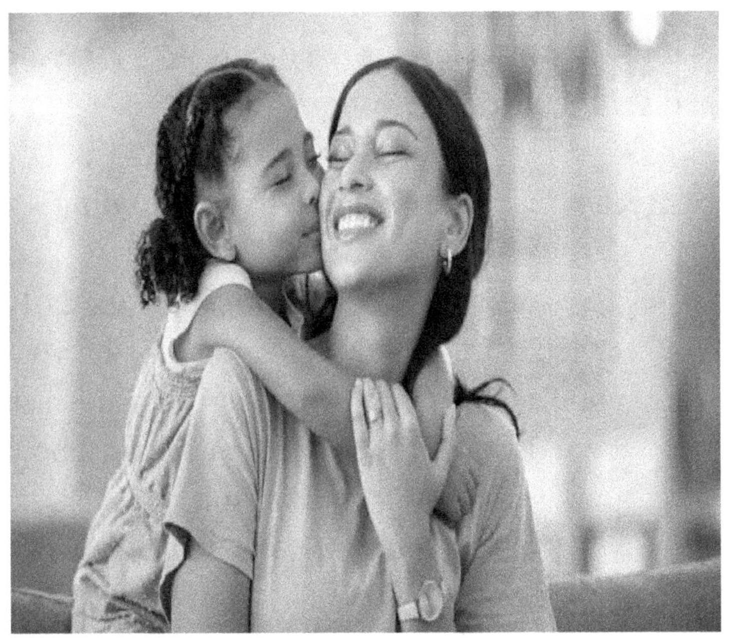

Even before your baby is born, a strong and life-changing attachment develops between parents and children. Understanding the value of early bonding and sustaining that bond are crucial for your child's emotional development as expectant parents. In this chapter, we'll look at ways to embrace the specialness of your parent-child relationship while creating a loving and secure bond with your infant.

A. Recognizing the Value of Early Bonding

- **The basis for trust and security:** Early attachment lays the groundwork for your child's perception of security and trust. Your baby may explore and learn about the world in a safe atmosphere thanks to your caring and responsive interactions with them.

- Early bonding is extremely important for influencing your child's brain development and emotional stability. You support the development of strong brain connections and emotional well-being by continuously attending to their needs and creating a loving atmosphere.

- **Creating a Lifelong Connection:** The foundation of your connection is the link you develop with your child in the early years. It creates a strong bond that will deepen and expand as your child grows.

B. Methods for Promoting a Secure and Loving Connection

- **Skin-to-Skin Contact:** Hold your infant up against your naked chest to benefit from the healing effects of skin-to-skin contact. It also helps to control their body temperature and releases hormones that make you and your baby feel happy.

- **Eye Contact and Responsive Communication:** Make frequent eye contact with your child and use responsive language when speaking to them. Their feelings and experiences are validated through this engagement, which promotes a sense of connection. Quickly attending to their wants and indications demonstrates your love and respect for them.

- **Gentle Touch and Cuddling:** By using gentle touch and cuddling, you may foster intimacy and connection. Physical touch, such hugging, gentle caresses, and massages, produces oxytocin and deepens your bond with your child.

- Explore the advantages of babywearing and kangaroo care, which involve holding your infant close to your body in a sling or carrier. These routines encourage parent-child relationships, provide you a sense of stability, and let you attend to your baby's needs while going about your everyday business.

C. Appreciating Your Parent-Child Relationship's Individuality

- **Celebrate Individuality:** Appreciate and highlight your child's special traits and personality. Encourage a sense of acceptance and love by embracing their uniqueness and allowing them the freedom to explore and express themselves.

- **Enjoy Shared Moments:** Cherish the time you spend with your infant. These shared activities, whether you're singing, reading, playing, or just watching them explore their environment, strengthen your relationship and generate enduring memories.

Being fully present and conscious is something you should work on when interacting with your child. Parent mindfully to foster greater understanding and connection by focusing your attention on the here and now without passing judgment.

Keep in mind that the relationship between a parent and child develops with time. You are building a foundation of love, trust, and security for your child by realizing the value of early bonding, using methods to create a loving connection, and accepting the particularities of your parent-child relationship.

Enjoy each moment and savor the strong link that is developing between you and your child as you start this amazing journey of parenthood. Their world will be shaped by your love and nurturing presence, which will build the foundation for a lifetime of adoration, kinship, and joy.

Here are some more tips and techniques to help you strengthen your relationship as you continue to build the parent-child bond:

- **Play is a strong tool for connecting and learning;** use it to your advantage by engaging in meaningful play. Play games that are age-appropriate and encourage conversation, exploration, and imagination. Get on the ground, follow your child's lead, and establish a loving, amusing environment for them to develop.

- Practice active listening by giving your child your full attention while keeping an open mind and heart. Recognize their verbal and nonverbal signs, affirm their sentiments, and react sympathetically. You may give your child a secure place to express themselves and strengthen your relationship of trust by actively listening to them.

- **Establish Rituals and Routines:** Give your child a sense of consistency and security by establishing rituals and routines. These can be straightforward daily routines like bedtime rituals, mealtime customs, or distinctive family traditions. These customs foster a sense of belonging and improve the link between parents and children.

- **Practice Positive Discipline:** Positive discipline focuses on teaching and guiding your child's conduct rather than punishing them. Employ positive discipline strategies that emphasize comprehension, empathetic behavior, and problem-solving. You may encourage a closer bond and assist your child in gaining self-control and emotional intelligence by creating a caring and respectful environment.

Remember to seek support and take care of yourself because sustaining the parent-child relationship also necessitates doing so. Join parenting organizations, ask for help from family members, or get in touch with experts who can provide you direction and assurance. It is possible to be totally present and emotionally accessible for your child when you look after your own well-being.

Celebrate the pleasures and difficulties that come with your parent-child connection as you embrace its singularity. Each parent-child relationship is unique and develops in its own manner. Accept the process of learning and development as you negotiate the complex dance of parenthood.

You have learnt the value of early bonding, methods for creating a warm relationship, and the significance of valuing your particular parent-child relationship in this chapter. By putting these ideas into practice, you are cultivating a relationship that will last and grow throughout your child's life.

The finest gifts you can give your child are your love, care, and presence as you set out on this incredible journey. Enjoy the moments, make enduring memories, and bask in the splendor of the relationship between a parent and kid.

CHAPTER 3

ACCESSING PERSONAL CHANGES

A great amount of physical and emotional change occurs throughout pregnancy. We will look at how to accept the bodily changes that happen during pregnancy in this chapter. We will travel this journey together, celebrating the amazing transformations, engaging in self-care for our physical wellbeing, and encouraging body positivity and self-acceptance.

A. Honoring the Amazing Changes that Take Place During Pregnancy

- **Embracing the Miracle of Life:** Pregnancy ushers in the amazing process of conception. Enjoy the miracle of your body as it nourishes and cares for your developing child. Consider the amazing resilience and strength that pregnancy has revealed in you.

- **Appreciating the Physical Changes:** Pregnancy causes your body to go through a number of physical changes, including weight increase, changes in breast size, and an expanding tummy. Accept these changes as evidence of the amazing process occurring inside of you and as proof of the strength of your body.

- **Developing a Bond with Your Baby:** Your body's physical changes serve as a constant reminder of the wonderful bond you have with your child. Savor the strong relationship that is developing between you and your child as you feel their movements and notice the changes in your body.

B. Self-care techniques for maintaining physical health

- **Prioritize Rest and Sleep:** Because of the increased demands pregnancy makes on your body, it's critical to give rest and good sleep first priority. Make sure your bedroom is cozy for sleeping and pay attention to your body's signals. Take brief rest periods throughout the day to refuel and revitalize.

- **Gentle Movement:** Take part in gentle movements and exercises that enhance physical wellbeing. Stretching, prenatal yoga, swimming, and walking can all help ease pain, boost circulation, and increase general strength and flexibility.

- Choose a balanced, healthy diet that promotes both your health and the growth of your child in order to nourish your body. Variety of fruits, vegetables, whole grains, lean meats, and water should all be consumed. For nutritional advice that is specific to you, speak with your doctor.

- Self-care rituals should be practiced. Treat yourself to self-care rituals that encourage relaxation and physical well-being. Take calming baths, treat yourself to mild massages, practice deep breathing techniques, and partake in enjoyable hobbies.

C. Embracing self-acceptance and body positivity

- **Change Your Perspective:** Adopt a loving and upbeat attitude toward your evolving body. Recognize that every physical change is a reflection of the amazing process of bringing life into the world and caring for it.

- **Focus on Health and energy:** Change your attention from your outward look to your body's health and energy. Embrace the fortitude and resiliency that enable you to carry and feed your child.

- Find positive and inspiring influences, such as encouraging friends, family, and online groups. Surround Yourself with

Supportive Voices. On your path, being surrounded by others who value body positivity and self-acceptance can inspire and motivate you.

- **Practice Positive Affirmations:** Use positive affirmations to strengthen your sense of self-love and appreciation for your evolving physique. Remind yourself of the amazing things your body is capable of and the beauty you possess.

Keep in mind that every pregnancy is different and that every body reacts to changes in a different way. Accept the physical changes as evidence of the remarkable adventure that is parenthood. You can move through this transition period with grace and assurance by engaging in self-care, taking care of your body, and building body positivity and self-acceptance.

Celebrate the amazing changes, respect your body, and treasure the wonderful experience of being pregnant. You deserve love and acceptance from both yourself and people around you because you are a beautiful, powerful person who deserves it. Remember that your body is a vehicle for life with remarkable power and resilience as you accept the physical changes.

Throughout this journey, give your body the respect and attention it deserves. Here are some extra activities to promote body positivity and enhance your physical well-being:

Invest in comfortable, maternity-friendly apparel that makes you feel good about yourself. Dress comfortably and express your personal style. Pick out outfits that let you show off your individual flair while accommodating your changing figure. Accept fashion as a means of self-expression in this unique period.

Consult with medical professionals that specialize in prenatal and postnatal care to get competent advice. They can offer advice on workouts, physical adjustments, and particular self-care techniques that are tailored to your need. Putting together a caring healthcare team will guarantee that you have the knowledge and experience necessary to take on this path with assurance.

Develop a deeper relationship with your body by engaging in mindful body awareness exercises. Spend some time tuning in to your body's movements, sensations, and alterations. Practice body scans and focused breathing to cultivate an attitude of gratitude and acceptance.

Document your pregnant journey with images or a journal to capture and celebrate it. Be sure to document your physical development and significant turning points. You can embrace pregnancy's transformational nature and recognize the beauty of your changing physical form by thinking back on these memories.

CHAPTER 4

GENERATING A SAFE AND NUTRITIOUS SETTLEMENT

A: Designing a Cozy and Friendly Space for Your Baby in Section

For your baby's comfort and growth, you must create a warm and friendly environment. The information in this area will help you build a nurturing atmosphere that supports your baby's health and happiness.

Creating a Nursery Floor Plan

Plan out your baby's nursery's layout first. Take into account the room's flow and how various spaces will be used. Make room for the crib, changing table, storage, and a comfortable lounging area where you may spend time with your child. Make sure the furniture is arranged such that it is accessible and easy to move about.

Selecting Calming Colors and Décor

Choose nursery furnishings and colors that promote a peaceful ambiance. Soft pastel colors like light blue, delicate pink, or mint green can help create a calming atmosphere. Create a calm and friendly environment for your infant by including natural elements, such as animal-themed wall art or patterns from nature.

Providing Furniture That Is Comfortable and Practical

For the nursery of your child, make an investment in cozy, practical furniture. Pick a crib with a comfortable mattress that complies with safety regulations. For feeding and cuddling sessions, think about a rocking or gliding chair. Choose a durable changing table that has room for plenty of diapers, wipes, and other necessities. Choose pieces of furniture that are simple to keep and clean.

Making a Sensory-Rich Setting

By including sensory-rich elements in the nursery, you can stimulate your baby's senses. To stimulate the sense of sight, use wall decals, soft toys, and mobiles. To improve their sense of touch, include soft blankets, textured rugs, and tactile toys. To create a pleasant auditory atmosphere, think about playing quiet music or relaxing sounds.

B: Practical Advice for Childproofing and Safety Measures

To protect your baby's safety as they explore their environment, you must childproof your home. The information in this part will help you build a safe atmosphere and stop accidents and injuries.

Make a thorough evaluation of your home's safety

Start by performing a complete evaluation of your home's safety. Determine any dangers that might exist, such as sharp edges, frayed cords, or unsteady furniture. Look out for electrical outlets, home chemicals that need to be stored safely, and choking dangers. You can prevent risks by taking proactive action by recognizing these threats.

Add locks and safety gates.

To avoid falls, place safety gates at the top and bottom of staircases. To keep potentially dangerous items and substances out of reach, install safety latches and locks on cupboards, drawers, and appliances. To prevent unintentional falls, lock or window-guard windows. The safety of your newborn can be greatly improved by taking these easy steps.

Child-safe electrical plugs and cords

To stop your baby from putting things in electrical outlets, cover them with outlet covers or safety plugs. To avoid trip risks or unintentional pulls, secure dangling cords and wires. To keep them out of your baby's grasp, use cord concealers or organizers. For increased convenience and security, think about installing outlet covers that slide shut automatically when not in use.

Anchor Heavy Items and Secure Furniture

To prevent tipping, fasten furniture like bookcases, dressers, and televisions to the wall. To hold heavier objects in place, use wall anchors or furniture straps. As infants start to pull themselves up and explore their environment, this precaution is essential. By securing furniture, accidents are avoided and their safety is guaranteed.

C: Creating a Peaceful Environment at Home

For your wellbeing as expectant parents and to build a loving environment for your child, creating harmony in your household is crucial. Insights and helpful advice on creating a harmonious environment at home that fosters a sense of calm, love, and connection are offered in this area.

Fostering Transparent Communication

The foundation of a peaceful home environment is open communication. Encourage your partner to have frank discussions with you about your feelings, thoughts, and goals for motherhood.

Talk about your parenting principles, objectives, and worries. Establish a secure environment where you may voice your opinions, listen intently, and discover points of agreement. As you set out on this adventure together, effective communication will help to develop trust and enhance your relationship.

Creating Customs and Rituals

You and your infant will feel more secure and predictable if you establish routines and rituals. Set up a consistent schedule for meals, bedtimes, and playtime. Routine consistency can provide your child a sense of security and contribute to a calm and happy home environment. Use traditions to develop connection and forge enduring memories, such as reading bedtime stories, singing lullabies, or sharing meals as a family.

Self-care and stress management techniques

A pleasant environment at home depends on you taking care of yourself. Self-care and stress management must be prioritized because parenting can be stressful. Find leisure pursuits that will relax and refresh you, such as exercise, meditation, or hobbies. Ask for help if you need it from friends and family and don't be afraid to do so. You'll be better able to give your infant a nurturing and loving atmosphere if you take care of your own well-being.

Creating a Positive and Loving Environment

By expressing love, thanks, and admiration for one another, you may create a pleasant and caring environment. Hugs, kisses, and cuddles are all effective ways to express love. Validate each other's feelings and experiences while engaging in active listening. Make your home a place where empathy, respect, and kindness are valued. You may lay the groundwork for both you and your child's mental well-being by cultivating a pleasant and supportive environment.

Conflict Resolution and Support-Seeking

Any partnership will inevitably experience conflicts, so it's critical to resolve them amicably. Use constructive conflict-resolution techniques including active listening, quietly expressing your emotions, and reaching compromises. If disputes linger or become out of hand, think about getting help from a therapist or counselor for couples. Don't be afraid to ask for help; qualified advice can help you overcome obstacles and improve your relationship.

Creating a Network of Support

Embrace a network of family, friends, and other parents who will support you. Through parenting clubs, internet forums, or regional community organizations, get in touch with other new or expectant parents. It can be really helpful to talk about your experiences, ask for guidance, and get support from others who are traveling a similar path. A robust network of supporters offers inspiration, compassion, and useful help, fostering a supportive environment for your family.

Keep in mind that fostering harmony at home is a continuous process that calls for effort, tolerance, and adaptability. Celebrate the love and connection that develops within your family, embrace the happy occasions, and work through the difficulties together.

CHAPTER 5

NEUTRALLY NEGOTIATING PRACTICALITIES

A: Budgeting for Your Growing Family and Financial Considerations

Planning and budgeting your finances carefully are essential while getting ready for a baby. To help you manage the financial aspects of starting a family and ensure long-term financial stability, this section will offer insights and useful advice.

Taking Stock of Your Financial Situation

Analyze your existing financial condition and consider how growing your family may affect it. Find out how to figure out your income, expenses, and debts. Learn how to make a realistic budget that takes the extra expenses of raising a child into account.

Preparing for healthcare costs and parental leave

Learn about your options for parental leave and the costs involved with taking time off from work. Examine several pregnancy, birth, and postpartum healthcare plans and coverage alternatives. Learn how to prepare and save for potential out-of-pocket expenses.

Saving for the future of your child

Learn the value of saving for your child's future needs, such as education and other long-term requirements. Investigate several savings choices, such as investment accounts and college funds. Learn how to make financial objectives, contribute consistently to savings, and take advantage of compound interest.

B: Organizing Baby Essentials and Developing a Sustainable Lifestyle

Organizing necessities and developing a sustainable lifestyle that is consistent with your values are important parts of being ready for the birth of your child. This section will offer helpful advice on setting up baby needs, implementing eco-friendly habits, and reducing trash.

Putting Together a Baby Registry and Checklist

Find out how to make a thorough baby registry and necessary checklist. Learn about the necessities for the birth of your child, including clothing, diapers, feeding equipment, and nursery furniture. Learn the advantages of choosing environmentally friendly and sustainable items, and look at the resources available for locating ethical and sustainable brands.

Managing and Organizing Baby Equipment

Learn how to manage and organize baby supplies to make the most of your available space. Learn how to organize your space and make storage options that work for your infant. Learn useful tips for preserving a clutter-free home while managing infant necessities such as clothing, toys, and other necessities.

Using sustainable methods and reducing waste

By adding eco-friendly habits into your daily routine, adopt a sustainable lifestyle. Learn about utilizing natural and organic infant care products, cloth diapering, and reducing the usage of single-use items. Learn how to reduce trash in your home and recycle, compost, and more.

Investigate environmentally friendly feeding techniques, such as breastfeeding and creating your own baby food.

C: Juggling Family and Work Life

The well-being of you and your family depends on achieving a healthy work-life balance. This section will offer tips for juggling job obligations with parenthood expectations, preserving your personal wellbeing, and fostering your family ties.

Having Conversations with Your Employer

Examine the best ways to express to your employer your wants and expectations. Find out about your entitlements and rights, such as maternity and paternity leave, flexible work schedules, and child care assistance. Learn how encouraging workplace environments may be created by using open and honest communication.

Prioritization and Time Administration

Learn time management strategies that work to balance your obligations to your family and your job. Study methods for allocating tasks according to importance, establishing rules, and assigning duties. Learn techniques for increasing productivity and efficiency so that you may spend quality time with your family and at work.

Family time that's good and self-care

Put your family's needs first and take care of yourself to keep a healthy work-life balance. Find family-friendly activities to engage in to make memorable memories. Discover the value of self-care and methods for incorporating self-care activities into your daily life.

Investigate your options for finding support, including family and friends, support groups, and outside assistance.

Every family's path is different, so it's important to identify strategies that suit your needs and circumstances. You may easily negotiate the realities of parenting and take pleasure in the process of expanding your family with careful preparation, organization, and a focus on keeping a healthy work-life balance.

CHAPTER 6

GETTING READY FOR ARRIVAL

A. Investigating Your Birth Options and Making a Birth Plan

It's essential to research your delivery options as you near the end of your pregnancy and to make a birth plan that reflects your preferences and aspirations. This chapter will walk you through the process, assisting you in making wise choices and getting ready for the birth of your child.

- **Knowing Your Birth alternatives:** There are a variety of birth alternatives accessible, from natural birth to painkiller medications. Spend some time learning about each choice, keeping in mind things like your health, the welfare of the infant, and any personal preferences you might have. Talk to your healthcare professional about your alternatives; they can offer insightful advice.

- **The process of writing a birth plan:** A birth plan is a written statement of your preferences and goals for the labor, delivery, and postpartum period. It acts as a channel of communication between you, your partner, and your medical staff. Start by going over the key components of your birth plan, such as how you want to manage pain, how you want to labor, how you want to be monitored, and whether you want any support people in the delivery room. Be flexible and aware that your birth plans may need to be modified depending on the situation.

- **Working Together with Your Healthcare Provider:** It's critical to work together with your healthcare provider after you have a general concept of your birth preferences. They can offer helpful insights, talk about any medical issues, and give suggestions on how to make your birth plan as thorough and practical as you can. By working together, you can be sure that your birth plan will be compatible with the facilities and medical knowledge at your disposal.

B. What to Bring for a Comfortable Stay in the Hospital

The process of getting ready for your hospital stay is thrilling because it signals that your baby's arrival is about to happen. The necessities you should bring will be explained in this part to help you have a relaxing and stress-free trip.

- Pack comfortable, loose-fitting clothing for your stay in the hospital, including pajamas, nursing bras, and cozy underwear. Bring a bathrobe, stockings, and slippers so you can move around more comfortably. Also think about bringing comforting and familiar items like a favorite pillow, blanket, or plush animal.

- Bring your necessary amenities, such as your toothbrush, toothpaste, shampoo, conditioner, soap, and any other preferred personal care products. Packing lip balm, moisturizer, and hair ties will help you stay fresh during your hospital stay.

- **Documentation and Important Information:** Make sure you bring all the required papers, such as identification, insurance information, and any essential hospital paperwork. A list of crucial phone numbers, such as those for your doctor, your family, and your friends who will be supporting you throughout this time, is also useful.

C. Accepting the Joy and Wonder of Having Your Baby

It's crucial to appreciate the excitement and wonder of welcoming your kid as the anticipation grows. This section will look at how to communicate with your expanding family and strengthen the emotional connection both before and after the baby is born.

- Take the time to capture this special time in your life's journey. Think about keeping a pregnancy journal or scrapbook where you may record milestones and express your emotions. To preserve these priceless experiences for future generations, you can also capture pictures or record films.

- **Nurture the Emotional Bond:** Engage in bonding activities with your infant to strengthen your relationship. Play relaxing music, softly massage your belly, and talk, sing, or read to your infant. These encounters not only foster a feeling of connection, but they also give your child a safe haven.

- **Share the Joy:** Include your spouse, your family, and your close friends in the process of having a baby. Plan a celebration or baby shower to honor the impending birth. This not only enables you to share the joy, but it also builds a network of family and friends who will be there to assist you both during and after the birth.

- **Attend Parenting programs:** Take a look at the seminars or programs that are being given in your area. These courses can offer helpful advice and knowledge on baby care, breastfeeding, infant CPR, and other crucial abilities. As you are ready to become parents, going to these seminars with your spouse can enhance your confidence and solidify your relationship.

- **Accept Self-Care:** During this stage, give self-care top priority. Spend some time unwinding, doing what makes you happy, and engaging in self-care rituals like yoga, meditation, or mild exercise. Keep in mind that caring for yourself is just as vital as caring for your child.

- Join Communities or Support organizations to Connect with Other expectant Parents: Look for communities or support organizations where you can join forces with other expectant parents. It may be incredibly comforting and encouraging to discuss experiences, worries, and suggestions with others who are traveling a similar path.

Finally, as you get ready for your baby's arrival, spend some time considering your birth alternatives and making a birth plan that fits your preferences. In addition to preparing for a peaceful hospital stay, you should also embrace the joy and wonder of having your new baby by documenting the experience, fostering your relationship with your partner, and involving your loved ones in the celebration. Do not forget to put self-care first and ask for assistance from communities of expectant parents. The birth of your child is a lovely and life-changing moment, and by mentally and emotionally preparing, you are laying the groundwork for a happy and fulfilling transition into parenthood.

CHAPTER 7

ENJOYING THE FIRST WEEK WITH A BABY

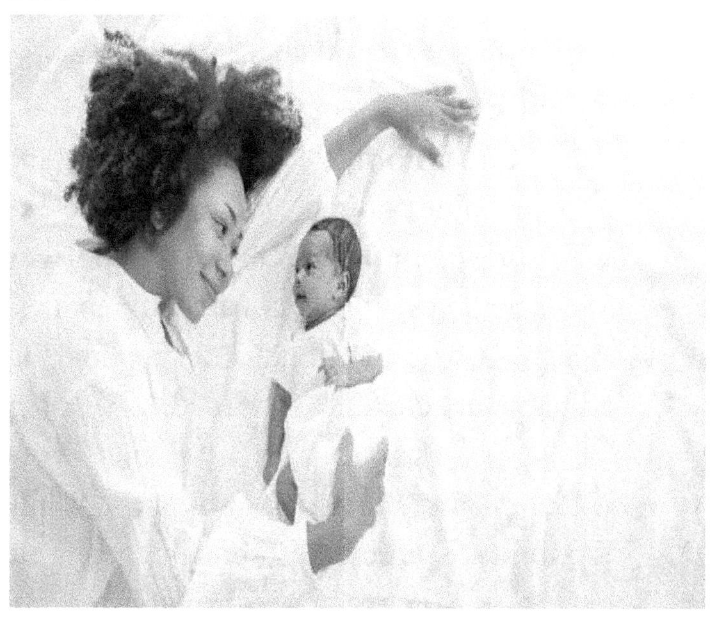

Spending the first few weeks with your newborn is invaluable and transformative. We'll look at how to navigate this period with grace and joy in this chapter, with a focus on adjusting to the new schedule and sleeping habits, fostering family time, and using loving care. We'll also emphasize how important it is to take care of oneself after giving birth and seek out support.

A: Acclimating to the New Routine and Sleeping Patterns

- **Accept Flexibility:** Be conscious of the unpredictable nature of the first few weeks with a newborn. Babies have certain needs and schedules that can vary day to day. Accept flexibility, and be prepared to adjust your schedule as needed.

- **Create a Simple pattern:** While flexibility is crucial, establishing a simple pattern can help you and your baby feel more secure and organized. Schedule everyday activities like tummy time and gentle play as well as regular feeding and sleep times. Be patient and give yourself and your kid enough time to become adjusted to the new rhythm. Routines take time to establish.

- **Prioritize Your Sleep:** Sleep deprivation can be a problem for new parents. Prioritize your sleep by resting when your child does, asking your partner or family members for help, and creating a sleep-friendly environment. Remember that your level of health will determine how well you can care for your baby.

B. Encouraging meaningful interactions and employing tact

- **Skin-to-Skin Contact:** Touch your baby's skin as much as you can. Improved nursing, bonding, and temperature and heart rate management are all benefits of this therapy. Take pleasure in the closeness and connection you get when holding your infant against your bare chest.

- Whether you choose to breastfeed or bottle-feed, these feeding times present fantastic opportunities for bonding. Make eye contact, create a calm and comfortable environment, and cherish these intimate moments when you can feed and cuddle with your child.

- To calm and relax your baby, look into soothing methods like infant massage and soft touch. Use gentle pressure and strokes to promote relaxation and relieve any discomfort or flatulence your baby may experience. Additionally, explore with various relaxing techniques like swaddling, rhythmic movement, or using white noise to create a calming and comforting environment.

C. Using self-compassion and getting help after giving birth

It is important to practice self-compassion because the postpartum period can be emotionally and physically exhausting. Work on this and be kind to yourself. Recognize that a range of emotions, including happiness, exhaustion, and vulnerability, are frequent. Give yourself permission to put your health first, to rest when you need to, and to ask for help.

Speak to your spouse, your family, and your friends to get their support. Allow them to share in the joy of parenting your child and be willing to accept their assistance. Their assistance, whether it be through household chore assistance, listening, or encouraging words, can be quite helpful during this time.

- **Join Support Groups:** Consider visiting postpartum support groups or socializing with other new parents in your community. These groups offer a safe environment where members may share experiences, obtain advice, and find comfort in the knowing that others are going through similar situations. Finding people who are interested in the same things as you could make you feel less alone and provide you access to a community that is supportive.

As you negotiate the joyful and challenging parts of raising a new baby, keep in mind that every parent and kid are unique. Give yourself permission to grow with your child and trust your instincts. Enjoy these wonderful weeks because they mark the beginning of a lifelong bond and the incredible journey that is parenthood.

By adjusting to the new routine and sleeping habits, encouraging bonding periods, and practicing self-compassion, you are laying the groundwork for a positive postpartum experience. As you embrace the joy, challenges, and chances for growth that come with caring for your new baby, be aware of your support network. This chapter has provided you with wise guidance to assist you in cherishing the first few weeks with your child. Take advantage of this unique time and cherish the memories you create.

CHAPTER 8

HONORING DEVELOPMENTAL MARKERS

Seeing your child develop and hit developmental milestones is a thrilling journey full of wonder and happiness. We'll look at ways to identify and encourage your baby's development in this chapter. We'll work hard to comprehend your child's developmental phases, take part in beneficial learning activities, and appreciate the individuality of your baby's journey.

A. Recognizing Your Baby's Growth and Developmental Stages

During the newborn stage, your baby is adjusting to life outside the womb. They are establishing relationships with their carers, strengthening their reflexes, and gaining sensory awareness. Make sure they are in a secure and comforting setting, attend to their needs very soon, and give them lots of skin contact.

- **Infant stage:** During this time, your infant begins to engage and move around more. They might even start to turn over and crawl as they spread their arms out and grab things. By allowing them to spend a lot of time on their stomachs, exercising moderately, and exposing them to appropriate objects and textures, you can promote their physical development.

- When your child reaches the toddler stage of development, their ability to communicate verbally, interact with others, and use their motor skills will all significantly advance. By providing a stimulating atmosphere, engaging toys and books, opportunities for investigation, and pretend play, you can pique children's curiosity.

B. Engaging in Activities That Are Meaningful and Promote Learning

Play with sensory toys to arouse your baby's senses. Provide them with textured objects and safe, age-appropriate toys so they may use their senses of touch, sight, sound, smell, and taste to discover the world around them. This promotes their mental and sensory growth as well as an inquisitive and investigative mentality.

- **Reading and storytelling:** From a young age, expose your child to the world of literature. Your baby's language skills will improve and your relationship with them will deepen as you read to and share stories with them. You may make reading a fun, creative activity by selecting books appropriate for your child's age that have vibrant illustrations and other interesting features.

- Encourage your child to enjoy music and physical activity. Play musical instruments, dance, and sing songs together. In addition to enhancing coordination, language abilities, and rhythm sense, music promotes cognitive maturation. Allow your infant to do moderate motions or exercises like baby yoga, and let them experiment with their own movements.

C. Consider Your Baby's Growth a Special Experience.

- **Avoid Comparisons:** It's best to avoid comparing the growth of your child to that of other children because every baby develops at a different rate. Pay attention to each person's unique skills and accomplishments as you accept and respect their journey. Keep in mind that every infant is different and develops at their own rate.

- Recognize and celebrate all of your child's accomplishments, no matter how minor. Each victory represents a crucial turning point in their development. Take the time to enjoy and document these special moments, whether it's their first grin, rolling over, or speaking.

The parent who best comprehends your child is you. The growth of your instinct and intuition depends on your ability to trust them. Recognize their cues, take note of their interests, and modify your interactions and activities to suit their particular requirements. Keep in mind that you are their best friend and compass.

Honoring your baby's developmental milestones is a rewarding journey that requires familiarity with the many growth and developmental phases, participation in significant projects, and acceptance of the individuality of their path. Enjoy the sweet moments as your child progresses through new developmental stages and welcome each one with love, patience, and attention. Remember that they will need your love and support to help them grow and develop. You may nurture your baby's potential and foster a setting that is helpful to their development by being aware of their developmental stages, engaging in learning-stimulating activities, and appreciating their individuality.

Be sure to capture and preserve these unique moments as you commemorate each milestone. To preserve the memories, take photographs, write in a journal, or put together a scrapbook. Think about how much and how far your child has come.

Most importantly, enjoy the journey. Being able to watch your child develop and grow is a luxury. Enjoy your child's progress in all of its wonder and excitement, and cherish the relationship you are building with them. As they develop into the wonderful person they were supposed to be, appreciate and celebrate their distinctiveness.

I'd like to say hello and congrats on finishing the first stage of parenthood. With your love, care, and dedication, you are giving your child the best foundation for a happy and fulfilling life. The future holds a plethora of opportunities. Keep track of your child's developmental milestones and relish watching them mature.

CHAPTER 9

CARE FOR YOUR PARTNERSHIP

Maintaining your relationship becomes increasingly important as you start your parenting adventure. This chapter will cover relationship building, effective communication, balancing parenting responsibilities, and cultivating moments of connection and delight.

A: Strengthening your bond as you begin parenthood is item number

Set quality time as a top priority by scheduling time exclusively for the two of you. Despite the rigors of parenting, it's crucial to retain a strong connection in your love relationship. Make time for one another by going on dates, spending quiet evenings together, or engaging in a common hobby.

- **Express Gratitude and Appreciation:** Set aside some time each day to express gratitude and appreciation to your partner. Recognize and appreciate what they have done as a parent and a partner. These modest acts of gratitude can deepen your relationship and create a welcoming environment.

- **Seek Support:** Keep in mind that you are a team and that asking for assistance is acceptable. Lean on one another and look for assistance from loved ones, friends, or support groups. You can overcome the difficulties and keep a strong relationship by splitting the duties of parenthood and supporting one another.

B. Parenting roles must be balanced while maintaining effective communication

- **Open and Honest Communication:** Good communication is essential to preserving a happy relationship. Establish a secure environment where you may freely share your ideas, worries, and demands. Actively hear what your partner has to say, acknowledge their emotions, and work together to come up with solutions that complement both of your parenting responsibilities.

- **Define and Assign Parenting Responsibilities:** Talk with your partner about and assign parenting responsibilities. Consider your unique strengths, hobbies, and work schedules to find a balance that works for you both. Finding a harmonic balance between your parenting duties requires being flexible and being transparent with one another.

Recognize that you and your partner may have different parenting philosophies and support one another's parenting approaches. Instead of seeing these distinctions as a point of contention, embrace them as a strength. Find areas of agreement when it comes to key choices affecting the raising of your child by supporting and respecting each other's views.

C. Fostering Connection and Shared Joy Moments

- **Establish Rituals That Foster Connection:** Create rituals that encourage kinship and delight. The activities can be as straightforward as eating dinner as a family, going on walks, reading bedtime stories together, or hosting a regular family game night. These customs provide you the chance to connect, make enduring memories, and solidify your family's foundation.

Together, you should celebrate your baby's milestones as well as your own as parents. As a team, recognize and honor accomplishments big and small. You strengthen your relationship and foster a healthy environment in your partnership by sharing these happy moments with one another.

- **Practice Gratitude:** Develop an attitude of gratitude in your marriage. Spend some time appreciating the little pleasures, the assistance you give one another, and the luxury of co-parenting. Gratitude expression strengthens your partnership and promotes positivity.

In conclusion, when you begin the road of motherhood, nurturing your relationship is crucial. You are creating a strong foundation for your family by enhancing your bond, developing efficient communication, choosing parental responsibilities that are balanced, and generating special moments of connection and delight. Don't forget to put your relationship first, to help one another out, and to share in the joys of parenthood. You are creating the foundation for a happy and fulfilling family life by developing your partnership, which is the center of a caring and nurturing environment for your child.

Keep in mind that your partnership is a source of strength and support as you negotiate the rewards and difficulties of motherhood. While it is common to encounter challenges along the way, by actively fostering your relationship, you can work through them as a couple.

Communicate honestly and openly, taking the time to comprehend one another's viewpoints and requirements. Find strategies to fairly divide parenting duties while taking into account each other's advantages and disadvantages. Accept the distinctiveness of your own parenting philosophies and work together to give your child the best care possible.

Prioritize times of connection and joy-sharing in the middle of parenting chaos. Make family ties and celebrations of milestones a part of your routines. These experiences not only solidify your relationship but also help you and your child develop enduring memories.

Do not forget to take care of yourself and give your partner space to rest. By looking after your own needs, you can be the best versions of yourselves for your child and for each other.

Finally, show each other patience and forgiveness. Making errors is part of learning to be a parent. Approach problems with empathy and a desire to solve them jointly. Your relationship is a journey, and you can face the joys and challenges of motherhood together if you have love, patience, and open communication.

Congratulations on reaching this point in your pregnancy journey. By fostering your relationship, you not only give your child a caring and encouraging environment, but you also lay the groundwork for a long-lasting union. Cherish the opportunities for development, joy, and connection that motherhood gives as you embark on the adventure ahead.

CHAPTER 10

PARENTS' SELF-CARE

Being a parent is wonderful and fulfilling, but it can also be difficult at times. It is imperative that you prioritize self-care and maintain your emotional wellbeing as you set out on this journey. This chapter discusses the value of self-care, coping mechanisms for parental stress and weariness, the efficacy of self-compassion, and how to ask for help when you need it.

A. Making self-care and emotional stability a top priority

It is not selfish to take care of your needs; rather, doing so is essential for your welfare and capacity to provide for your child. Identify Your Needs: Realize that attending to your needs is not being selfish. Recognize your everyday physical, emotional, and mental requirements and attend to them.

- **Create Clear Boundaries:** Create clear boundaries to safeguard your time and energy. When you have too many responsibilities and chores, learn to say no. The things that make you joyful and give you energy should take precedence.

- **Exercise in Self-Reflection:** Give yourself some time to reflect on and comprehend who you are. Check in with yourself frequently to determine your needs and emotional state. You can learn to understand and manage your emotions by keeping a journal, practicing meditation, or simply spending some time alone.

B. Techniques for Dealing with Parental Stress and Tiredness

Get in touch with your network of supporters if you need help. Ask your partner, your family, your friends, or online parenting communities for assistance when you need it. Stress can be reduced and helpful support can be given by dividing the workload.

Use breathing and mindfulness exercises: Include breathing and mindfulness practices in your everyday routine. You can release tension, find inner peace, and refuel by practicing deep breathing techniques, following a guided meditation, or partaking in activities like yoga or nature excursions.

Time management and organization: To lessen emotions of burden, use efficient time management techniques and organizational frameworks. Establish routines, assign duties to others, and prioritize chores to give your day-to-day existence some structure and balance.

C. Increasing Self-Compassion and Seeking Assistance When Required

By accepting self-compassion, one can be patient and understanding with oneself. Recognize that as a parent, you're doing the best you can. By granting yourself forgiveness, letting go of perfectionism, and accepting the ups and downs of parenthood as a process, you may embrace self-compassion.

Don't be afraid to seek professional assistance if you are struggling with chronic stress, anxiety, or postpartum depression. Counselors, therapists, or support groups that focus on parental mental health may be helpful when help is needed.

find other parents who can connect to your difficulties and make friends with them. Join parenting seminars, discussion boards, or support groups for parents. Sharing your struggles and successes with others who share your interests can make you feel accepted and validated.

Keep in mind that you will be better equipped to care for your child if you take care of yourself. To preserve emotional well-being when parenting, it's important to prioritize self-care, use coping skills, and practice self-compassion.

Congratulations on beginning the amazing road that is parenthood. By investing in your personal health, you can create a positive atmosphere for both you and your child. When you need help, rely on your network of friends and family, and remember that looking after yourself is an act of love for both you and your family. Consider every day a chance for development, and treasure the joy and connections that parenthood gives.

Remember to practice self-care as you go further down your parenting path; it is a lifelong endeavor. The following suggestions are presented to help you with your emotional health and self-care:

- **Develop Your Hobbies and Interests:** Schedule time for the pursuits that make you feel content and happy. Self-indulgence is beneficial for your general health, whether it comprises hobbies, creative endeavors, sports, or physical routines.

- Make Eating Wholesome Foods, Regular Exercise, and Getting Enough Sleep a Priority: Establish these healthy living practices to make eating Whole Foods, Regular Exercise, and Getting Enough Sleep a Priority. You'll be able to handle the difficulties of parenthood more successfully if you have a healthy, energized physique.

- **Parent with self-compassion:** Treat yourself with the same respect and tolerance as you would your child. Recognize your shortcomings and be kind to yourself. Remember that raising a child is a learning process in which you advance alongside them.

- **Create Alone Time:** Block off some time to think and recharge. By engaging in activities like writing, solitary tea breaks, or nature walks, you can reconnect with yourself. These peaceful moments can revitalize you and open your eyes to fresh perspectives.

- **Keep the lines of communication open with your partner:** Discuss your needs, worries, and feelings with them constantly. Your partnership will be bolstered by effective communication that fosters mutual support. You can control your stress and keep a balance in your lives by cooperating to discover solutions.

Spend some time reflecting on the benefits and joys of becoming a parent as a self-reflection and gratitude exercise. You can record incidents of admiration and thanks in a gratitude diary. You can lift your spirits and develop a sense of fulfillment by thinking back on the good things that have happened along the way as a parent.

Self-care is not a luxury but a necessity. You are modeling perseverance and good habits for your child by putting your health first. As you navigate the delicate complexity of parenthood, have an open mind to the path of personal growth. As long as you continue to take care of yourself and your child, you deserve to be treated with respect, compassion, and support.

Thank you for reading "Anticipating the Journey: Insights for Expecting Parents." I wish you happiness, love, and close bonds with your child on your journey.

CONCLUSION

Take a minute as you finish reading this booklet, "Anticipating the Journey: Insights for Expecting Parents," to consider the life-changing trip you are about to go on. You can now add priceless insights and information to the anticipation and excitement you felt at the beginning of this book, which will help you navigate the lovely complexity of parenthood.

A. Examining the Life-Changing Experience of Becoming a Parent

Being a parent transforms you, reshaping your priorities, values, and sense of self. This journey has been filled with emotions, amazement, and anticipation from the moment you first saw the miracle of new life developing inside of you to the eagerness to meet your lovely baby. While you are getting ready to welcome your child into the world, take the time to respect and enjoy this transforming journey.

B. Lasting Inspiration and Nurturing Support

It's crucial to keep in mind that you are not alone as you enter the world of parenthood. Although having children might be difficult, it is also incredibly gratifying. Enjoy the peace of mind that comes from knowing that you have the knowledge and resources you need to successfully complete this adventure. Accept the ups and downs with open minds and hearts, understanding that every event is an opportunity for development, education, and strengthening your relationship with your child.

You are strong, adaptable, and full of love. As you manage the joys and challenges that lie ahead, trust your instincts, ask for help when you need it, and be kind to yourself and your partner. Never forget to put yourself last, care for your relationship, and build a group of people who support you.

C: Resources for Additional Reading and Getting Involved in Supportive Communities

You now have a solid foundation of knowledge thanks to this ebook, but there is always more to discover. Consider learning more about particular interests as you progress in becoming a parent. The following resources can be used to read more and find helpful communities:

- Explore a range of parenting and child development books that are tailored to your individual needs and interests as parents. There is a lot of information out there that is just waiting to be explored, from baby care to gentle parenting techniques.

- Parenting websites, social media groups, and online forums are great places to meet other parents. These groups offer a forum for exchanging stories, getting suggestions, and getting support from those who can identify with your path.

- Consider signing up for parenting seminars or workshops that are being offered in your neighborhood. These tools offer practical advice, transferable skills, and a chance to physically interact with other parents.

- **Parenting Support Groups:** Look for local parenting support groups where you can connect with other parents facing comparable difficulties. These organizations provide a supportive environment where members can talk about their experiences, get advice, and get support from those who have gone through motherhood themselves and can relate.

Just keep in mind that this is only the beginning of your adventure. New milestones, experiences, and discoveries will be revealed every day. As parents, embrace the wonder, the difficulties, and most importantly, the love that will define your lives.

Congratulations on achieving this important life milestone. You are ready to start the amazing path of motherhood with love, patience, and the knowledge you have received. May you spend each day with your child sharing love, laughter, and special memories. Take in the experience, treasure the memories, and relish each moment of this wonderful journey that is motherhood.